दत्तात्रेय योगशास्त्र

Dattātreya Yogaśāstra

(English Translation Accompanied by Sanskrit
Text in Roman Transliteration)

Translated into English by
Swami Vishnuswaroop

Published by

Divine Yoga Institute

Kathmandu, Nepal

Dedication

This book is dedicated to my Guru Swami Satyananda Saraswani,

Founder of Bihar School of Yoga,

Munger, India.

Contents

Dedication...iii

Gratitude... v

Introduction 1

Dattātreya Yogaśāstra 3

A Key to Transliteration 63

Also by This Author... 65

Gratitude

First of all I would like to express my heartfelt salutations to Adinatha (the Primordial Master) and my Guru Swami Satyananda Saraswati for their unwavering inspiration and guidance I have received for my work. I realize that my firm faith and belief in God and Guru is a motivational gift for me in completing this work. I could never have done it without their blessings.

I am always thankful to Ms. Bhawani Uprety for her untiring support she has provided me during my involvement in writing and translating various classical texts on yoga. My due thanks goes to her forever.

On the occasion of the Guru Purnima Day I wish that may God and Guru inspire us to tread the path of yoga in order to achieve the ultimate goal of human life!

- Swami Vishnuswaroop

Introduction

Dattātreya Yogaśāstra, in a dialogue form between *Sānkriti* and Lord *Dattātreya*, is a unique classical yogic text. It imparts the right concept and rational knowledge of yoga with a heavy focus on practice with great effort. It clearly outlines that everyone is entitled to yoga practice regardless of one's age, sex, faith and belief, sect and cult and tradition and religion, and robe and physical appearance.

Regarding the four stages of yoga, the text mentions *ārambha, ghaṭa, paricaya* and *niṣpatti avasthās*. On the practices of the *Haṭhayoga*, it elaborates mainly eight *bandhas* and *mudrās* which are *mahamudra, mahabandha, khecari mudrā, jāladhara, uddiyāna* and *moola bandhas, viparitakar ana* and *vajroli*.

Of *yamas* and *niyamas* the *Yogaśāstra* regards that eating less (*laghvahara*) and *ahimsā* are supreme respectively. Of all the asanas, practice of *padmāsana* alone is highly recommended and also regarded as the destroyer of all diseases.

The *Yogaśāstra* emphasizes that one can not achieve success in yoga just by reading scriptures, by wearing special garbs/dresses, by repeating mantras and by worshiping Gods and deities, but by constantly practicing it without sloth.

Dattātreya Yogaśāstra regards *prāṇāyāma* as an important practice in yoga *sādhanā*. *Padmāsana* is highly recommended for the practice of *prāṇāyāma*.

The techniques of *prāṇāyāma* are fully elaborated with the inclusion of the practice of three *bandhas* and *sahita kumbhaka* (with the retention of breath) for the purification of *nāḍis*. It is further described that when the *nāḍis* are purified, the signs of success in the body of yogi become visible. When *kumbhaka* practice is prolonged gradually every day, the yogi finally attains *kevala kumbhaka* that is the ultimate goal of *prāṇāyāma* practice.

The text also explains that when *kevala kumbhaka* is achieved, the yogi experiences several signs in his body and attains some minor *siddhis*. This is called the *ārambha avasthā* (stage). When *kevala kumbhaka* is perfected through further practice, he attains *ghaṭa avasthā*. This is a very important stage in which *prāna* and *apāna, manas* and *prāṇa* and *ātmā* and *paramātmā* are united. It instructs further that the yogi in this stage should practice *pratyāhāra*. While practicing *pratyāhāra*, the yogi feels unity will one and all and also he attains miraculous powers, but he is advised neither to be attached to them nor to disclose them.

The text further elaborates that when perfection is attained through practice on five elements, the yogi attains supernatural powers like *anima,* etc. Then the yogi should continue his practice of meditation first on *saguṇa brahma* and then *nirguṇa brahma* so he can finally attain the culmination of yoga, *nispatti avasthā* in which he realizes the union with God. After achieving his union with God, at this stage, the yogi as per his wish may leave his body or he may wander as a *jīvan mukta* (one who is liberated while living) in this universe.

Publisher

Dattātreya Yogaśāstra

दत्तात्रेय योगशास्त्र

Salutation to Nṛsiṁha

नृसिंहरूपिणे चिदात्मने सुखस्वरूपिणे ।

पदैस्त्रिभिः तदादिभिः निरूपिताय वै नमः ॥१॥

nṛsiṁharūpiṇe cidātmane sukhasvarūpiṇe /

padaistribhiḥ tadādibhiḥ nirūpitāya vai namaḥ /1/

Salutations to the one who has the form of *Nṛsiṁha* (the incarnation of *Viṣṇu*), whose consciousness is the Self, whose form is of bliss, and who is described by the three words, i.e. *Saccidanānda* (*sat, cit* and *ānanda*). -1.

Sāṅkṛti Arrives at Naimiṣāraṇya

साङ्कृतिर्मुनिवर्योऽसौ भूतये योगलिप्सया ।

सकलं भूः परिभ्राम्यन् नैमिषारण्यमाप्तवान् ॥२॥

sāṅkṛtirmunivaryo'sau bhūtaye yogalipsayā /

sakalaṃ bhūḥ paribhrānyan naimiṣāraṇyamāptavān /2/

Sāṅkṛti, the best of *munis*, after roaming the whole earth in the hope of acquiring (knowledge of) yoga, arrived at the forest called *naimiṣāraṇya*. -2.

सुगन्धिनानाकुसुमैः स्वादुसत्फलसंयुतैः ।

शाखिभिः शोभितम् पुण्यं जलकासारमण्डितम् ॥३॥

sugandhinānākusumaiḥ svādusatphalasaṃyutaiḥ /

śākhibhiḥ shobhitaṃ puṇyaṃ jalakāsāramaṇḍitam /3/

The forest was decorated with various flowers of good fragrance, the branches of the trees with delicious fruits and ponds of water in it. -3.

Sāṅkṛti Meets Mahāmuni Dattātreya

स मुनिर्विचरम्स्तत्र ददर्शाम्रतरोरधः ।

वेदिकायां समासीनं दत्तात्रेयं महामुनिम् ॥४॥

बद्धपद्मासनासीनं नासाग्रार्पितया दृशा ।

ऊरुमध्यगतोत्तानमणियुग्मेन शोभितम् ॥५॥

saḥ munirvicaraṃstatra dadarśāmrataroradhaḥ /

vedikāyāṃ samāsīnaṃ dattātreyaṃ mahāmunim /4/

baddhapadmāsanāsīnam nāsāgrārpitayā dṛśā /

ūrumadhyagatottānamaṇiyugmena śobhitam /5/

The *Muni* (*Sāṅkṛti*) while roaming there suddenly met *Mahāmuni* (the great sage) *Dattātreya*, sitting on a pedestal under a mango tree in a bound-lotus pose gazing on the tip of his nose, adorned with his hands joined together on his lap. -4-5

तत: प्रणम्यमखिलं दत्तात्रेयं महामुनिम् ।

तच्छिष्यै: सह तत्रैव सम्मुखश्चोपविष्टवान् ॥६॥

tataḥ praṇamyamakhilaṃ dattātreyaṃ mahāmunim /

tacchiṣyaiḥ saha tatraiva sammukhaścopaviṣṭavān /6/

Then, *Sāṅkṛti* sincerely saluted the *Mahāmuni Dattātreya* and sat down there with his pupils facing towards him. -6.

Lord Dattātreya Welcomes Sāṅkṛti

तदैव स मुनिर्योगात् विरम्य स्वपुर: स्थितम् ।

उवाच सांकृतिं प्रितिपूर्वकं स्वागतं वच: ॥७॥

tadaiva sa muniryogāt viramya svapuraḥ sthitam /

uvāca Sāṅkṛtim pritipūrvakam svāgataṃ vacaḥ /7/

At that time the *Mahāmuni* came out of his deep-rooted yoga *sādhanā* and saw *Sāṅkṛti* at his place and spoke to him loving and welcoming words. -7.

Sāṅkṛti Questions on Yoga

साङ्कृते कथय त्वं मां किमुद्दिश्य इहागत: ।

इति पृष्टस्तु स प्राह योगं ज्ञातुमिहागत: ॥८॥

sāṅkṛte kathaya tvam mām kimuddiśya ihāgataḥ /

iti pṛṣṭastu sa prāha yogam jñātumihāgataḥ /8/

The *Mahāmuni* said, "*Sāṅkṛti*, tell me with what purpose you have come here." After he was asked this question, he replied that he had come to him to obtain the knowledge of yoga. -8.

Lord Dattātreya Answers on Yoga

योगो हि बहुधा ब्रह्मन् तत्सर्वं कथयामि ते ।

मन्त्रयोगो लयश्चैव हठयोगस्तथैव च ।

राजयोगश्चतुर्थः स्यात् योगानामुत्तमस्तु सः ॥९॥

आरम्भश्च घटश्चैव तथा परिचयः स्मृतः ।

निष्पत्तिश्चेत्यवस्था च चतुर्थी परिकल्पिता ।

एतेषां विस्तरं वक्ष्ये यदि त्वं श्रोतुमिच्छसि ॥१०॥

yogo hi bahudhā brahman tatsarvaṃ kathayāmi te /

mantrayogo layaścaiva haṭhayogastathaiva ca /

rajayogaścaturthaḥ syāt yogānāmuttamastu saḥ /9/

ārambhaśca ghaṭaścaiva tathā paricayaḥ smṛtaḥ /

niṣpattiścetyavasthā ca caturthī parikalpitā /

eteṣāṃ vistaraṃ vakṣye yadi tvaṃ śrotumicchasi /10/

Mahāmuni Dattātreya said: - O *Brahman*! There are many forms of yoga. I will describe all of them to you. They are *Mantrayoga, Layayoga, Haṭhayoga* and the fourth is *Rājayoga* which is the best of all yogas. It is said that there are four stages of yoga. They are *ārambha, ghaṭa, paricaya* and the fourth is *niṣpatti*. I will explain to you in detail if you wish to hear about them. -9-10.

Dattatreya Yogashastra

Mantrayoga Practice

अङ्गेषु मातृका न्यासपूर्वं मन्त्रं जपन्सुधीः ।

यं कञ्चनाभिसिद्ध्यै स्यान्मन्त्रयोगः स कथ्यते ॥११॥

aṅgeṣu mātṛkā nyāsapūrvaṃ mantraṃ japansudhīḥ /

yaṃ kacanābhisiddhyai syānmantrayogaḥ sa kathyate /11 /

First of all, the wise man should recite a mantra after placing the *mātṛkās* (the alphabets) on his bodily parts. It is called *Mantrayoga* which can be perfected by everyone. -11.

Mantra Sidddhi in Twelve Years

मृदुस्तस्याधिकारी स्याद्द्वादशाब्दैस्तु साधनात् ।

प्रायेण लभते ज्ञानं सिद्धिश्चैवाणिमादिकाः ॥१२॥

mṛdustasyādhikārī syāddvādaśābdaistu sādhanāt /

prāyeṇa labhate jñānaṃ siddhiścaivāṇimādikāḥ /12/

A mild *sādhaka* (pratitioner) who is entitled to practice it can attain *jñāna* (knowledge, wisdom) probably after twelve years of practice in addition to *siddhis* (perfections) like *aṇimā*, etc. -12.

Mantrayoga as Lower Practice

अल्पबुद्धिरिमं योगं सेवते साधकाधमः ।

मन्त्रयोगो ह्ययं प्रोक्तो योगानामधमस्तु सः ॥१३॥

alpabuddhirimaṃ yogaṃ sevate sādhakādhamaḥ /

mantrayogo hyayaṃ prokto yogānāmadhamastu saḥ /13/

A *sādhaka* (spiritual pratitioner) who is inferior and has a low level of intellect serves (performs) this yoga. Of all the yogas, *Mantrayoga* is called the lowest one. -13.

Layayoga Practice and Its Saṅketas

लययोगश्चित्तलयः सङ्केतैस्तु प्रजायते ।

आदिनाथेन सङ्केता अष्टकोटिः प्रकीर्त्तिताः ॥१४॥

layayogaścittalayaḥ saṅketaiḥ tu prajāyate /

ādināthena saṅketā aṣṭakoṭi prakīrttitāḥ /14/

Layayoga is the yoga of dissolution of the mind. It occurs through various *saṅketas* (points/ places/ methods of concentration). *Ādinātha* has revealed eighty million *saṅketas* for dissolution. -14.

Sāṅkṛti Questions on Ādinātha

साङ्कृतिरुवाच ।

भगवन्नादिनाथस्सः किं रूपः कः सः उच्यताम् ।

Sāṅkṛtiruvāca:

bhagavannādināthaḥ saḥ kiṃ rūpaḥ kaḥ saḥ ucyatām /15/

Sāṅkṛti said: "Please tell me, what type of form does *Ādinātha* has? Who is he?" -15.

Dattātreya Answers his Question

दत्तात्रेय उवाच ।

महादेवस्य नामानि आदिनाथादिनकान्यपि ।

शिवेश्वरश्च देवोऽसौ लीलया व्यचरत्प्रभुः ॥१५॥

dattātreya uvāca:

mahādevasya nāmāni ādināthādinakānyapi /

śiveśvaraśca devo'sau līlayā vyacaratprabhuḥ /15 /

*Dattā*treya said: "The names of *Mahādeva* are *Ādinātha*, *Bhairava*, *Śiveśvara* and *Deva* during the time when the Lord was involved in his pastimes". -16.

Ādinātha's Places of Pastimes

श्रीकण्ठपर्वते गौर्या सह प्रमथनायकान् ।

हिमाक्षपर्वते चैव कदलीवनगोचरे ॥१६॥

śrīkaṇṭhaparvate gauryā saha pramathanāyakān /

himākṣaparvate caiva kadalīvanagocare /16 /

His places of pastimes with *Pārvatī* accompanied by the leaders of his troop were on top of Mount *Śrīkaṇṭha* and Mount *Himākṣa* and in the vastness of the banana forest. -16.

Lord Śaṅkara tells on Varied Saṅketas

गिरिकूटे चित्रकूटे सुपादपयुते गिरौ ।

कृपयैकैकसङ्केतं शङ्करः प्राह तत्र तान् ॥१७॥

girikūṭe citrakūṭe supādapayute girau /

kṛpayaikaikasaṅketaṃ śaṅkaraḥ prāha tatra tān /17/

On the mountain of *Citrakūṭa* surrounded with magnificent forests, Lord *Śaṅkara* with his due kindness spoke the *saṅketa* (method of dissolution) in each of those places there. -17.

Saṅketas are Innumerable

तानि सर्वाणि वक्तुं हि न शक्नोमि तु विस्तरात् ।

कानिचित्कथयिष्यामि सहजाभ्यासवत्सुखम् ॥१८॥

tāni sarvāṇi vaktum tu na hi śaknomi vistarāt /

kānicitkathayiṣyāmi sahajābhyāsavatsukham /18 /

I cannot describe all of them elaborately. I am going to tell you some of them which are natural and comfortable to put into practice. -18.

Meditation on Śūnya, Sole Saṅketa

तिष्ठन् गच्छन्स्वपन्भुञ्जन् ध्यायन्शून्यमहर्निशम् ।

अयमेको हि संकेतः आदिनाथेन भाषितः ॥१९॥

tiṣṭhan gacchansvapanbhuñjan

dhyāyanśūnyamaharniśam /

ayameko hi saṅketaḥ ādināthena bhāṣitaḥ /19/

While sitting, going/moving, sleeping, eating throughout the day and night one should meditate on *śūnya* (void). This is one of the saṅketas (methods) alone taught by *Ādinātha*. -19.

Alternative Saṅketa – Nosetip Gazing

नासाग्रदृष्टिमात्रेण अपरः परिकीर्तितः ।

शिरः पश्चाच्च भागस्य ध्यानं मृत्युं जयेत् परम् ॥२०॥

nāsāgradṛṣṭimātreṇa aparaḥ parikīrtitaḥ /

śiraḥ paścācca bhāgasya dhyānam mṛtyum jayet param /20 /

Alternative method of practice taught is simply gazing at the tip of the nose. By the meditation on the hind part of the head, one grandly conquers death. -20.

Alternative Saṅketa – Eyebrow Center Gazing

भूमध्यदृष्टिमात्रेण परः सङ्केतः उच्यते ।

ललाटे भूतले यश्च उत्तमः सः प्रकीर्तितः ॥२१॥

bhrūmadhyadṛṣṭimātreṇa paraḥ saṅketaḥ ucyate /

lalāte bhrūtale yaśca uttamaḥ saḥ prakīrtitaḥ /21/

Another method of practice highly spoken is simply gazing at the eyebrow center. Gazing at the spot between the two eyebrows on the forehead is said to be magnificent. -21.

Alternative Saṅketa – Big Toes Gazing

सव्य दक्षिण पादस्य अङ्गुष्ठे लयमुत्तमम् ।

उत्तानशववत्भूमौ शयनं चोक्तमुत्तमम् ॥२२॥

savya dakṣiṇa pādasya aṅguṣṭhe layamuttamam /

uttānaśavavatbhūmau śayanam coktamuttamam /22/

One excellent practice of *laya* (dissolution) is gazing at the big toes of the left and right feet. Lying down on the ground facing upward like a dead person is also called an excellent (practice of) *laya* (dissolution). -22.

Practice in a Solitary Place

शिथिलो निर्जने देशे कुर्यात् चेत्सिद्धिमाप्नुयात् ।

एवं च बहुसङ्केतान् कथयामास शङ्करः ॥२३॥

śithilo nirjane deśe kuryāt cetsiddhimāpnuyāt /

evaṃ ca bahu saṃketān kathayāmāsa śaṅkaraḥ /23/

If practiced in a solitary place in a relaxed way, success will be attained. In this way, many methods of laya have been spoken by *Śaṅkara*. -23.

Many Other Saṅketas Exist

सङ्केतैः बहुभिश्चान्यैः यस्य चित्तलयो भवेत् ।

स एव लययोगः स्यात् कर्मयोगं ततः श्रणुः ॥२४॥

saṅketaiḥ bahubhiścānyaiḥ yasya cittalayo bhavet /

sa eva layayogaḥ syāt haṭhayogaṃ tataḥ śṛṇuḥ /24/

Cittalaya (dissolution of the mind) that happens with those *saṅketas* (methods of concentration mentioned above) and other methods of dissolution are already (practices of) *Layayoga* (the Yoga of Dissolution). After it, listen (to me) about *Karmayoga* (here it means *Aṣṭāṅgayoga*, the yoga of eight limbs). -24.

Description of Karmayoga

यमश्च नियमश्चैव आसनं च ततः परम् ।

प्राणायामश्चतुर्थः स्यात् प्रत्याहारस्तु पञ्चमः ।

ततस्तु धारणा प्रोक्ता ध्यानं सप्तममुच्यते ॥२५॥

yamaśca niyamaścaiva āsanaṃ ca tataḥ param /

prāṇāyāmaścatuthaḥ syāt pratyāhārastu pañcamaḥ /

tatastu dhāraṇā proktā dhyānaṃ saptamamucyate /25/

Yama (rules) and niyama (restraints) are supreme and then there is asana (a pose/posture); *prāṇāyāma* (breathing methods/techniques) is the fourth, *pratyāhāra* (withdrawal of the senses) is the fifth. Then next is called *dhāraṇā* (concentration) and *dhyāna* is the seventh. -25.

Karmayoga Also Known as Aṣṭāṅgayoga

समाधिः अष्टमः प्रोक्तः सर्वपुण्यफलप्रदः ।

एवमष्टाङ्गयोगं च याज्ञवल्क्यादयो विदुः ॥२६॥

samādhiḥ aṣṭamaḥ proktaḥ sarvapuṇyapradaḥ /

evamaṣṭāṅgayogaṃ ca yājñavalkyādayo viduḥ /26/

Samādhi (the superconscious state) is said to be the eighth limb (the last one) which bestows the highest merits of all. Thus, *aṣṭāṅgayoga* (the eight limbs or parts of yoga) are known by the wise sages like *Yājñavalkya* and others. -26.

Haṭhayoga Mudrās and Bandhas

कपिलाद्यास्तु शिष्याश्च हठं कुर्युस्ततो यथा ।

तद्यथा च महामुद्रा महाबन्धस्तथैव च ॥२७॥

ततः स्यात्खेचरीमुद्रा बन्धो जालन्धरः तथा ।

उड्डियाणं मूलबन्धो विपरीतकरणी तथा ॥२८॥

kapilādyāstu śiṣyāśca haṭhaṃ kuryustato yathā /

tadyathā ca mahāmudrā mahābandhastathaiva ca /27/

tataḥ syātkhecarīmudrā bandho jālandharaḥ tathā /

uḍḍiyāṇaṃ mūlabandho viparītakaraṇī tathā /28/

Sage like *Kapila* and others, and their disciples practiced *Haṭhayoga* in their own way. It is like this: *mahāmudrā, mahābandha*; and then *khecarīmudrā* and *jālandhara bandha*; *uḍḍiyāṇa bandha, mūlabandha* and *viparītakaraṇī*. -27-28.

Vajroli and Amaroli Practices

वज्रोलिरमरोलिश्च सहजोलिस्त्रिधा मता ।

एतेषां लक्षणं वक्ष्ये कर्त्तव्यं च विशेषतः ॥२९॥

vajroliramaroliśca sahajolistridhā matā /

eteṣāṃ lakṣaṇaṃ vakṣye kartavyaṃ ca viśeṣataḥ /29/

Vajroli is thought to have three parts including *amaroli* and *sahajoli*. I am going to tell you about their characteristics and specifically, how they should be practiced. -29.

Of Yamas and Niyamas, Two Are Prime

यमा ये दश सम्प्रोक्ताः ऋषिभिः तत्त्वदर्शिभिः ।

लघ्वाहारस्तु तेष्वेको मुख्यो भवति नापरे ।

अहिंसा नियमेष्वेका मुख्या भवति नापरे ॥३०॥

yamā ye daśa samproktāḥ ṛṣibhiḥ tattvadarśibhiḥ /

laghvāhārastu teṣveko mukhyo bhavati nāpare /

ahiṃsā niyameṣvekā mukhyā bhavati nāpare /30/

[14]

The sages and those who saw the nature of the reality have spoken about ten *yamas*. Of them, *laghvāhāra* (*laghu* – little, *āhāra* – food, eating little or small amount of food) is principal and not others. Of *niyamas*, *ahiṃsā* (non-violence) is prime and not others. -30.

Of the Eighty-four Lākha Āsanas, The Best One

चतुरशीतिलक्षेषू आसनेषूत्तमं श्रृणु ।

आदिनाथेन सम्प्रोक्तं यद् आसनमिहोच्यते ॥३१॥

caturaśītilakṣeṣū āsaneṣūttamaṃ śṛṇu /

ādināthena samproktaṃ yad āsanamihocyate /31/

Of the eighty-four *lākha* (84,00,000) āsanas, hear about the best one, now the asana which is highly spoken by *Ādinātha* is described (below). -31.

Padmāsana Practice

उत्तानौ चरणौ कृत्वा उरुसंस्थौ प्रयत्न तहः ।

उरुमध्ये तथोत्तानौ पाणी कृत्वा ततो दृशौ ॥३२॥

नासाग्रे विन्यसेद् राजदन्तमूलं च जिह्वया ।

उत्तभ्य चिबुकं वक्षः संस्थाप्य पवनं शनैः ॥३३॥

यथाशक्ति समाकृष्य पूरयेदुदरं शनैः ।

यथाशक्त्यैव पश्चात्तु रेचयेत् पवनं शनैः ॥३४॥

uttānau caraṇau kṛtvorūsaṃsthau prayatnataḥ /

urū madhye tathottānau pāṇī kṛtvā tato dṛśau /32/

nāsāgre vinyased rājaddantamūlaṃ ca jihvayā /

uttabhya cibukaṃ vakṣaḥ saṃsthāpya pavanaṃ śanaiḥ /33/

yathāśakti samākṛṣya pūrayedudaraṃ śanaiḥ /

yathāśaktyeiva paścāttu recayet pavanaṃ śanaiḥ /34/

Turn both the feet upwards and cautiously place them on the opposite thighs. Place the hands on each lap and similarly turn them upwards. Gaze on the tip of the nose, insert the tongue into the throat pit, place the chin on the chest, inhale slowly according to capacity and slowly fill the abdomen. Then slowly exhale the air according to capacity. -32-34.

Padmāsana, Destroyer of All Diseases

इदं पद्मासनं प्रोक्तं सर्वव्याधिविनाशनम् ।

दुर्लभं येन केनापि धीमता लभ्यते भुवि ॥३५॥

idaṃ padmāsanaṃ proktaṃ sarvavyādhivināśanam /

durlabhaṃ yena kenāpi dhīmatā labhyate bhuvi /35/

This is called *padmāsana*. It destroys all diseases and it is rare to get it. It is accomplished by the wise men alone in this world. -35.

The Sequence of Yogic Practice

साङ्कृते श्रृणु सत्त्वस्थो योगाभ्यासक्रमं यथा ।

वक्ष्यमाणं प्रयत्नेन योगिनां सर्वलक्षणैः ॥३६॥

sāṅkṛte śṛṇu sattvastho yogābhyāsakramaṃ yathā /

vakṣyamāṇaṃ prayatnena yogināṃ sarvalakṣaṇaiḥ /36/

Sānskṛti, listen persistently to the sequence of yogic practice with due effort to be mentioned hereafter for all yogis with its all qualities. -36.

All Can Achieve Success in Yoga

युवावस्थोऽपि वृद्धो वा व्याधितो वा शनै: शनै: ।

अभ्यासात्सिद्धिमाप्रोति योगे सर्वोऽप्यतन्द्रितः ॥३७॥

yuvāvastho'pi vṛddho vā vyādhito vā śanaiḥ śanaiḥ /

abhyāsātsiddhimāpnoti yoge sarvo'pyatandritaḥ /37/

People who are in young stage or old or diseased, all can achieve success in yoga through practice without lassitude. -37.

ब्राह्मण: श्रमणो वा बौद्धो वाप्यार्हतोऽथवा ।

कापालिको वा चार्वाकः श्रद्धया सहितः सुधीः ।

योगाभ्यासरतो नित्यं सर्वसिद्धिमवाप्नुयात् ॥३८॥

brāhmaṇaḥ śramaṇo vā bauddho vāpyārhato'thavā /

kāpāliko vā cārvākaḥ śraddhayā sahitaḥ sudhīḥ /

yogābhyāsarato nityaṃ sarvasiddhimavāpnuyāt /38/

Whether a *Brāhmaṇa* or an ascetic or a *Buddhist* or a *Jain* or a *Kāpālika* (skull holder) or a *Cārvāka* (an eastern materialist or the follower of *Cārvāka*), a wise man with due faith through his constant devoted yogic practice gains all perfections. -38.

Perfection through Practice Alone

क्रियायुक्तस्य सिद्धि: स्यादक्रियस्य कथं भवेत् ।

न शास्त्रपाठमात्रेण काचित्सिद्धिः प्रजायते ॥३९॥

kriyāyuktasya siddhiḥ syādakriyasya katham bhavet /

na śāstrapāṭhamātreṇa kācitsiddhiḥ prajāyate /39/

Siddhi (perfection) is gained by one who is actively involved in (yogic) practices. How can it happen for one who does not practice? *Siddhi* does not occur just by mere reading or studying *śāstras* (the scriptures). -39.

Practice Alone Matters, Not the Garbs and Cults

मुण्डितो दण्डधारी वा काषायवसनोऽपि वा ।

नारायणवदो वापि जटिलो भस्मलेपनः ॥४०॥

नमः शिवायवाची वा बाह्यार्चा पूजकोऽपि वा ।

द्वादशस्थानपूजो वा बहुवत्सलभाषितम् ।

क्रियाहीनोऽथवा कूरः कथं सिद्धिमवाप्नुयात् ॥४१॥

muṇḍito daṇḍadhārī vā kāṣāyavasano'pi vā /

nārāyaṇavado vāpi jaṭilo bhasmalepanaḥ /40/

namaḥ śivāyavācī vā bāhyārcā pūjako'pi vā /

dvādaśasthānapūjo vā bahuvatsalabhāṣitam /

kriyāhīno'thavā krūraḥ katham siddhimavāpnuyāt /41/

One who is *muṇḍito* (shaven-headed), or *daṇḍadhārī* (bearing a stick) or wearing an ochre dress; or one who says, '*Nārāyaṇa*', or one who has knotted hair or one who has smeared ashes (on his body), or one who says, '*Namaḥ Śivāya*', or one who worships external statues/idols; or one who worships at the twelve places of pilgrimage, or one who speakes loving and kind words: (none of the above states matters at all) if one does not actively practice or if one is cruel, how does one attain *siddhi* (perfection)? -40-41.

Grace of God through Practice

न वेषधारणं सिद्धे: कारणं न च तत्तथा ।

कृपैव कारणं सिद्धे: सत्यमेव तु साङ्कृते ॥४२॥

na veṣadhāraṇaṃ siddheḥ kāraṇaṃ na ca tattathā /

kṛpaiva kāraṇaṃ siddheḥ satyameva tu sāṅkṛte /42/

Siddhi (perfection) cannot be attained by wearing robes, nor it can be the cause of it. Grace of God or *Guru* through practice alone is the cause of *siddhi* (perfection). *Sāṅkṛti*, this is certainly true. -42.

Yogic Story Tellers Deceive People

शिश्रोदरार्थं योगस्य कथया वेषधारिण: ।

अनुष्ठानविहीना: तु वञ्चयन्ति जनान्किल ॥४३॥

śiśnodarārthaṃ yogasya kathayā veṣadhāriṇaḥ /

anuṣṭhānavihīnāḥ tu vañcayanti janānkila /43/

It is said that men who wear religious garbs and tell the story of yoga for the enjoyment of foods and drinks, and those who do not practice of religious austerities, they only deceive people. -43.

उच्चावचै: विप्रलंभै: यतन्ते कुशला: नरा: ।

योगिनो वयमित्येवं मूढा: भोगपरायणा: ॥४४॥

uccāvacaiḥ vipralambhaiḥ yatante kuśalāḥ narāḥ /

yogino vayamityevaṃ mūḍhāḥ bhogaparāyaṇāḥ /44/

Cunning men make efforts for various types of deception and declare that they are yogis. They are nothing, but fools engaged in sensual pleasure. -44.

Discarding Men without Practice

शनैस्तथाविधान् ज्ञात्वा योगाभ्यासविवर्जिताम् ।

कृतार्थान्वचनैरेव वर्जयेद्द्वेषधारिणः ॥४५॥

śanaistathāvidhān jñātvā yogābhyāsavivarjitām /

kṛtārthānvacanaireva varjayedveṣadhāriṇaḥ /45/

Slowly when it becomes known that men who think that they achieve their goal only through words without practise of yoga, such men just wearing religious garbs (without practice and knowledge) should be abandoned. -45.

एते तु विघ्नभूतास्ते योगाभ्यासस्य सर्वदा ।

वर्जयेत्तान् प्रयत्नेन ईदृशी सिद्धिदा क्रिया ॥४६॥

ete tu vighnabhūttāste yogābhyāsasya sarvadā /

varjayettān prayatnena īdṛśī siddhidā kriyā /46/

These (people) are always obstacles to yogic practice. They should be visibly discarded with due efforts. Action like this bestows perfection. -46.

Obstacles in Yogic Practice

प्रथमाभ्यासकाले तु प्रवेशस्तु महामुने ।

आलस्यं प्रथमो विघ्नो द्वितीयस्तु प्रकथ्यते ।

पूर्वोक्तधूर्त्तगोष्ठी च तृतीयो मन्त्रसाधनम् ॥४७॥

prathamābhyāsakāle tu praveśastu mahāmune /

ālasyaṃ prathamo vighno dvitīyastu prakathyate /

pūrvoktadhūrttagoṣṭhī ca tṛtīyo mantrasādhanam /47/

O Great Sage! While entering into the practice for the first time, laziness is the first obstacle, the second is association with fraudulent people just described above and the third is the practice of mantras. – 47.

चतुर्थो धातुवादः स्यात् पञ्चमः खाद्यवादकम् ।

एवं च बहवो दृष्टाः मृगतृष्णाः समाः मुनेः ॥४८॥

caturtho dhātuvādaḥ syāt pañcamaḥ khādyavādakam /

evaṃ ca bahavo dṛṣṭāḥ mṛgatṛṣṇāḥ samāḥ muneḥ /48/

The fourth is alchemy and the fifth is enjoyment of pleasing foods and drinks. O Sage! There are various types of obstacles like mirage are seen. -48.

Removing Obstacles by Prāṇāyāma Practice

स्थिरासनस्य जायन्ते तां तु ज्ञात्वा सुधीः त्यजेत् ।

प्राणायामं ततः कुर्यात्पद्मासनगतः स्वयम् ॥४९॥

sthirāsanasya jāyante tāṃ tu jñātvā sudhīḥ tyajet /

prāṇāyāmaṃ tataḥ kuryātpadmāsanagataḥ svayam /49/

The wise man having established in his steady āsana (pose) should recognize those (obstacles) and shun them. Then he should practice *prāṇāyāma* in his *padmāsana*. -49.

Preparation of a Maṭha

सुशोभनं मठं कुर्यात्सूक्ष्मद्वारं तु निर्घुणम् ।

सुष्ठु लिप्तं गोमयेन सुधया वा प्रयत्न तः ॥५०॥

suśobhanaṃ maṭhaṃ kuryātsūkṣmadvāraṃ tu nirghuṇam /

suṣṭhu liptaṃ gomayena sudhayā vā prayatnataḥ /50 /

A beautiful hut with a small door should be made and it should be free of insects. It should be excellently made of clay and smeared with cow dung with due effort. -50.

मत्कुणैः मशकैः भूतैः वर्जितं च प्रयत्न तः ।

दिने दिने सुसम्मृष्टं सम्मार्जन्या ह्यतन्द्रितः ।

वासितं च सुगन्धेन धूपितं गुग्गुलादिभिः ॥५१॥

matkuṇaiḥ maśakaiḥ bhūtaiḥ varjitaṃ ca prayatnataḥ /

dine dine susammṛṣṭaṃ sammārjanyā hyatandritaḥ /

vāsitaṃ ca sugandhena dhūpitaṃ guggulādibhiḥ /51/

It should be carefully made free of bugs, mosquitoes and other creatures. It should be properly cleaned every day without laziness, perfumed with good fragrance and smoked with the *guggula* (commiphora wightil – botanical name) and others ((prescribed barks, branches, leaves and flowers of) trees and plants. -51.

मलमूत्रादिभिर्वर्गैरष्टादशभिरेव च ।

[22]

वर्जितं द्वारसम्पन्नम् ॥५२॥

वस्त्रं वाऽजिनमेव वा ।

नान्यत्र स्तरणासीनः परसंसर्गवर्जितः ॥५३॥

malamūtrādibhirvargairaṣṭādaśabhireva ca /

varjitaṃ dvārasampannam /52/

vastraṃ vā'jinameva vā /

nānyatra staraṇāsīnaḥ parasaṃsargavarjitaḥ /53/

The hut should be free from the eighteen types of impurities such as feces, urine and so on. It should have a door or cover with a cloth and the range of area should be free from grass and association of the public. –52-53.

Kumbhaka Practice in Padmāsana

तस्मिन् स तु समास्तीर्य आसनं विस्तृतांशकम् ।

तत्रोपविश्य मेधावी पद्मासनसमन्वितः ॥५४॥

tasmin sa tu samāstīrya āsanaṃ vistṛtāṃśakam /

tatropaviśya medhāvī padmāsanasamanvitaḥ /54/

There (in that hut), the wise yogi should extend his seat covered with a cloth and he should assume *padmāsana* (lotus pose). -54.

समकायः प्राञ्जलिश्च प्रणम्य स्वेष्टदेवताम् ।

ततो दक्षिणहस्तस्य अङ्गुष्ठेन इव पिङ्गलाम् ॥५५॥

निरुध्य पूरयेद् वायुमिडया च शनैः शनैः ।

यथाशक्तिनिरोधेन ततस्कुर्यात्तु कुम्भकम् ॥५६॥

samakāyaḥ prāñjaliśca praṇamya sveṣṭadevatām /

tato dakṣiṇahastasya aṅguṣṭhen iva piṅgalām /55/

nirudhya pūrayed vāyumiḍayā ca śanaiḥ śanaiḥ /

yathāśaktinirodhena tataskuryāttu kumbhakam /56/

With his body upright, he should salute his deity with his both hands joined together. Then he should close the right nostril with the right hand thumb and inhale slowly through the left nostril controlling the breath comfortably according to his capacity and then he should do *kumbhaka* (retention of the breath). -55-56.

ततस्त्यजेत्पिङ्गलया शनैः पवनवेगतः ।

पुनः पिङ्गलयाऽऽपूर्य पूरयेदुदरं शनैः ।

यथा त्यजेत्तथा तेन पूरयेदनिरोधतः ॥५७॥

tatastyajetpiṅgalayā śanaiḥ pavanavegataḥ /

punaḥ piṅgalayā''pūrya pūrayedudaraṃ śanaiḥ /

yathā tyajettathā tena pūrayedanirodhataḥ /57/

Then he should exhale the air through right nostril slowly without force. Again, he should inhale through right nostril and fill the abdomen slowly. Holding the breath as long as comfortable, he should gently exhale through the left nostril. Inhalation and exhalation should be performed in the same manner without interruption. -57.

Freedom from All Kinds of Planetary Effects/Evils

एवं प्रातः समासीनः कुर्याद् विंशति कुम्भकान् ।

कुम्भकः सहितो नाम सर्वग्रहविवर्जितः ॥५८॥

evaṃ prātaḥ samāsīnaskuryādviṃśatikumbhakān /

kumbhakaḥ sahito nāma sarvagrahavivarjitaḥ /58/

He should practice twenty *kumbhakas* performing the posture as per the aforesaid manner in the morning. This is called *sahita kumbhaka* which gives freedom from all kinds of planetary effects or all kinds of planetary obstacles/evils. -58.

Four Times a Day Practice

एवं मध्याह्नसमये कुर्यात् विंशतिकुम्भकान् ।

एवं सायं प्रकुर्वीत पुनः विंशतिकुम्भकान् ।

एवमेवार्धरात्रेऽपि कुर्यात् विंशतिकुम्भकान् ॥५९॥

evaṃ madhyāhnasamaye kuryāt vimśatikumbhakān /

evaṃ sāyaṃ prakurvīta punaḥ vimśatikumbhakān /

evamevārdharātre 'pi kuryāt vimśatikumbhakān /59/

In the same manner the *sahita kumbhaka* should be practiced twenty times in the midday, and again twenty times in the evening and also twenty times at midnight. -59.

कुर्वीत रेचपूराभ्यां सहितान्प्रतिवासरम् ।

सहितो रेचपूराभ्यां तस्मात् सहितकुम्भकः ॥६०॥

kurvīta recapūrābhyāṃ sahitānprativāsaram /

sahito recapūrābhyāṃ tasmāt sahitakumbhakaḥ /60/

It should be practiced with *recaka* (exhalation) and *pūraka* (inhalation) everyday. As it is practiced with *recaka* and *pūraka,* so it is called *sahita kumbhaka.* -60.

Purification of Nāḍīs in Three Months

कुर्यादेवं चतुर्वारमनालस्यो दिने दिने ।

एवं मासत्रयं कुर्यान्नाडीशुद्धिस्ततो भवेत् ॥६१॥

kuryādevaṃ caturvāramanālasyo dine dine /

evaṃ māsatrayaṃ kuryānnāḍīśuddhistato bhavet /61/

This *prāṇāyāma* should be practiced four times everyday without laziness for three months. Then all the *nāḍīs* (*prāṇic* pathways/ channels) will be purified. -61.

Signs of Purification of Nāḍīs

यदा तु नाडीशुद्धिः स्यात्तदा चिह्नानि बाह्यतः ।

जायन्ते योगिनो देहे तानि वक्ष्याम्यशेषतः ॥६२॥

yadā tu nāḍīśuddhiḥ syāttadā cihnāni bāhyataḥ /

jāyante yogino dehe tāni vakṣyāmyaśeṣataḥ /62/

When the *nāḍīs* are purified, these external signs will appear in the body of the yogi. I will describe all of them. -62.

शरीरलघुता दीप्तिः जठराग्निविवर्धनम् ।

कृशत्वं च शरीरस्य तदा जायेत्त निश्चितम् ॥६३॥

śarīralaghutā dīptiḥ jaṭharāgnivivardhanam /

kṛśatvaṃ ca śarīrasya tadā jāyetta niścitam /63/

Lightness and radiance in the body, increse of digestive fire and leanness of the body are certain to occur. -63.

Forbidden Things for Removing Obstacles

तदा वर्ज्यानि वक्ष्यामि योगविघ्नकराणि तु ।

लवणं सर्षपञ्चाम्लमुष्णं रूक्षं च तीक्ष्णकम् ॥६४॥

tadā varjyāni vakṣyāmi yogavighnakarāṇi tu /

lavaṇaṃ sarṣapañcāmlamuṣṇaṃ rūkṣaṃ ca tīkṣṇakam /64/

Then, I will describe all the causes that generate obstacles to yoga and those should be avoided. They are salt, mustard, foods that are sour and hot, and which give heating effect (in the body) and that are harsh (dry) and sharp. -64.

अतीव भोजनं त्याज्यं स्त्रीसङ्गमनमेव च ।

अग्निसेवा तु सन्त्याज्या धूर्त्तगोष्ठिश्च सन्त्यजेत् ॥६५॥

atīva bhojanam tyājyaṃ strīsaṅgamanameva ca /

agnisevā tu santyājyā dhūrtagoṣṭiśca santyajet /65/

Overindulging in foods and association with women (for sensual pleasure) should surely be avoided. *Agnisevā* (literally, service to fire, i.e. warming up with fire) should be avoided and also meetings with rogues should be avoided completely. -65.

Means of Gaining Success in Yoga

उपायं च प्रवक्ष्यामि क्षिप्रं योगस्य सिद्धये ।

घृतं क्षीरं च मिष्टान्नं मिताहरश्च शस्यते ॥६६॥

upāyaṃ ca pravakṣyāmi kṣipram yogasya siddhaye /

ghṛtaṃ kṣīraṃ ca miṣṭhānnaṃ mitāhāraśca śasyate /66/

Now I will tell you the means of gaining quick success in yoga. Butter, milk, sweet foods and *mitāhāra* (moderation in diet or moderate eating) are recommended. -66.

पूर्वोक्तकाले कुर्वीत पवनाभ्यासमेव च ।

ततः परं यथेष्टं तु शक्तिः स्याद् वायुधारणे ।

यथेष्टं धारणाद् वायोः सिध्येत्केवलकुम्भकम् ॥६७॥

pūrvoktakāle kurvīta pavanābhyāsameva ca /

tataḥ paraṃ yatheṣṭaṃ tu śaktiḥ syād vāyudhāraṇe /

yatheṣṭaṃ dhāraṇādvāyoḥ sidhyetkevalakumbhakam /67/

He should practice *prāṇāyāma* at the previously mentioned times (four times a day/twenty rounds). Then he will gain the ability to retain the breath inside as long as he desires. Through gaining the mastery over the retention of breath as long as he wishes, perfection in *kevala kumbhaka* (spontaneous retention of breath) will be achieved. -67.

Nothing Rare through Kevala Kumbhaka

केवले कुम्भके सिद्धे रेचपूरकवर्जिते ।

न तस्य दुर्लभं किञ्चित् त्रिषु लोकेषु विद्यते ॥६८॥

kevale kumbhake siddhe recapūrakavarjite /

na tasya durlabhaṃ kiñcit triṣu lokeṣu vidyate /68/

When perfection is attained in *kevala kumbhaka* without exhalation and inhalation, there is nothing impossible or rare for him in all the three worlds. -68.

Achievement of Dardurī Siddhi

प्रस्वेदो जायते पूर्वं मर्दनं तेन कारयेत् ।

ततोऽतिधारणाद् वायोः क्रमेणैव शनैः शनैः ॥६९॥

कम्पो भवति देहस्यासनस्थस्य योगिनः ।

ततोऽधिकतराभ्यासाद् दर्दुरी जायते धुवम् ॥७०॥

prasvedo jāyate pūrvaṃ mardanaṃ tena kārayet /

tato'ptidhāraṇād vāyoḥ krameṇaiva śanaiḥ śanaiḥ /69/

kampo bhavati dehasyāsanasthasya yoginaḥ /

tato'dhiratarābhyāsād dardurī jāyate dhruvam /70/

Perspiration starts first while practicing *kevala kumbhaka*. It should be rubbed on the body. Then if the retention of breath continued slowly in successive order, the yogi's body seated in āsana starts trembling. Through its continued further practice, *dardurī siddhi* (power to jump like a frog) is certainly achieved. -69-70.

यथा तु दर्दुरो गच्छेदुत्प्लुत्योत्प्लुत्य भूतले ।

पद्मासनस्थितो योगी तथा गच्छति भूतले ॥७१॥

yathā tu darduro gacchedutplutyotplutya bhūtale /

padmāsanasthito yogī tathā gacchati bhūtale /71/

Just like a frog jumps up and down on the ground, similarly the yogi sitting in *padmāsana* moves on the ground. -71.

Power to Levitate Through Kumbhaka

ततोऽधिकतराभ्यासाद् भूमित्यागश्च जायते ।

पद्मासनस्थ एवासौ भूमिमुत्सृज्य वर्त्तते ॥७२॥

निराधारोऽपि चित्रं हि तदा सामर्थ्यमुद्भवेत् ।

स्वल्पं वा बहु वा भुक्त्वा योगी न व्यथते तदा ॥७३॥

tato'dhikatarābhyāsād bhūmityagaśca jāyate /

padmāsanastha evāsau bhūmimutsṛjya varttate /72/

nirādhāro'pi citraṃ hi tadā sāmarthyamudbhavet /

svalpaṃ vā bahu vā bhuktvā yogī na vyathate tadā /73/

Then practicing the *kumbhaka* further, levitation arises. The yogi sitting in *padmāsana* remains raising (his body) off the ground without any support. Manifold powers bcome visible in him. The yogi does not suffer at all by eating a little bit or a lot. -72-73.

Decrese of Urine, Faeces and Sleep

अल्पमूत्रपुरीषस्तु स्वल्पनिद्रश्च जायते ।

क्रिमयो दूषिका लाला स्वेदो दुर्गन्धिता तनोः ।

एतानि सर्वदा तस्य न जायन्ते ततः परम् ॥७४॥

alpamūtrapurīṣastu svalpanidraśca jāyate /

krimayo dūṣikā lālā svedo durgandhitā tanoḥ /

etāni sarvadā tasya na jāyante tataḥ param /74/

His urine, faeces and sleep are decreased. Thereafter, worms, impurities of eyes, dripping of saliva, sweats and odour of the body all these never arise in his body. -74.

Achievement of Bhūcara Siddhi

ततोऽधिकतराभ्यासाद् बलमुत्पद्यते भृशम् ।

येन भूचरसिद्धिः स्याद् भूचराणां जये क्षमः ॥७५॥

tato'dhikatarābhāsād balamutpadyate bhṛśam /

yena bhūcarasiddhiḥ syād bhūcarāṇāṃ jaye kṣamaḥ /75/

Thereafter, by practicing further a great strength arises through which *bhūcara siddhi* is attained. He gains the power to win over all animals on earth. -75.

Power to Knock Down Animals

व्याघ्रो लुलायो वन्यो वा गवयो गज एव वा ।

सिंहो वा योगिना तेन म्रियन्ते हस्तताडनात् ।

कन्दर्पस्य यथारूपं तथा तस्यापि योगिनः ॥७६॥

vyāghro lulāyo vanyo vā gavayo gaja eva vā /

siṃho vā yoginā tena mriyante hastatāḍanāt /

kandarpasya yathārūpaṃ tathā tasyāpi yoginaḥ /76/

The tigers, buffalos, elephants, wild bulls and lions are killed by the blow of the hands of the yogi. His appearance becomes similar to *Kandarpa* (the god of love). -76.

Obstacle Due to Yogi's Loving Appearance

तस्मिन्काले महाविघ्नो योगिनः स्यात्प्रमादतः ।

तदूपवशगाः नार्यः काङ्क्ष्न्ते तस्य सङ्गमम् ॥७७॥

tasmin kāle mahāvighno yoginaḥ syātpramādataḥ /

tadrūpavaśagāḥ nāryaḥ kaṅkṣante tasya saṅgamam /77/

At that time, the yogi may face a great obstacle due to his negligence. Women, having infatuated by his handsomeness, desire to have sexual union with him. -77.

Avoiding the Company of Women

यदि सङ्गं करोत्येष बिन्दुस्तस्य विनश्यति ।

आयुः क्षयो बिन्दुनाशादसामर्थ्यं च जायते ।

तस्मात् स्त्रीणां सङ्गवर्जं कुर्यादभ्यासमादरात् ॥७८॥

yadi saṅgaṃ karotyeṣa bindustasya vinaśyati /

āyuḥ kṣayo bindunāśādasāmarthyaṃ ca jāyate /

tasmāt striṇām saṅgavarjaṃ kuryādabhyāsamādarāt /78/

If he is involved in sexual intercourse with them and his *bindu* (seminal fluid) is lost, his strength is destroyed and his life span is shortened. Therefore, he should give up the company of women and should go on performing his practice with due respect. -78.

Constant Preservation of the Bindu

योगिनोऽङ्गे सुगन्धिः स्यात् सततं बिन्दुधारणात् ।

तस्मात्सर्वप्रयत्नेन बिन्दुरक्ष्यो हि योगिना ॥७९॥

yogino'nge sugandih syāt satatam bindudhāraṇāt /

tasmātsarvaprayatnena binduraksyo hi yoginā /79/

A nice odour comes out of the body of the yogi through continuous *bindu dhāraṇā* (retention of semial fluid). Therefore, he should make all possible efforts in order to preserve his *bindu.* -79.

Pranava Destroys All Sins and Obstacles

ततो रहस्युपाविष्टः प्रणवं प्लुतमात्रया ।

जपेत्पूर्वार्जितानां च पापानां च नाशहेतवे ।

सर्वविघ्नहरश्चायं प्रणवः सर्वदोषहा ॥८०॥

tato rahasyupāviṣṭaḥ praṇavaṃ plutamātrayā /

japetpūrvārjitānāṃ ca pāpānāṃ ca nāśahetave /

sarvavighnaharaścāyaṃ praṇavaḥ sarvadoṣahā /80/

Then, remaining in a solitary place he should repeat the *pranava* (the mono syllable OM) following *plutamātrā* (chanting it by prolonging its duration three times) in order to destroy all the previously accumulated sins. This is the *pranava* which destroys all obstacles and eliminates all faults (on the path of yoga). -80.

Occurace of Arambha and Ghaṭa Stages

एवमभ्यासयोगेन सिद्धिरारम्भसम्भवा ।

ततो भवेद् घटावस्था पवनाभ्यासिनः सदा ॥८१॥

evamabhyāsayogena siddhirārambhasambhavā /

tato bhaved ghaṭāvasthā pavanābhyāsinaḥ sadā /81/

Through the practice of yoga (so far discoursed), the yogi can possibly attain the perfection of *ārambha* (*avasthā*) the beginning (stage). Then through constant practice of *kevala kumbhaka,* there arises *ghaṭa avasthā* (the vessel or the second stage). -81.

प्राणापानौ मनोवायू जीवात्मपरमात्मनौ ।

अन्योन्यस्याविरोधेन एकतां घटते यदा ।

तदा घटाद्वयावस्था प्रसिद्धा योगिनां स्मृता ॥८२॥

prāṇāpānau manovayū jīvātmaparamātmanau /

anyonyasyāvirodhenaikatāṃ ghaṭato kānicit /

tadā ghaṭādvayāvasthā prasiddhā yogināṃ smṛtā /82/

When the *prāṇa* and *apāna, manas* and *vāyu, ātmā* and *paramātmā* are united without any contradiction between the two (one another), then there arises *ghaṭa avasthā* which is declared by the famous yogis. -82.

ततश्चिह्नानि यानि स्युः तानि वक्ष्यामि कानिचित् ।

पूर्वं यः कथितोऽभ्यासश्चतुर्धा तं परित्यजेत् ॥८३॥

दिवा वा यदि वा रात्रौ याममात्रं समभ्यसेत् ।

एक बारं प्रतिदिनं कुर्यात् केवलकुम्भकम् ॥८४॥

tataścihnāni yāni syuḥ tāni vakṣyāmi kānicit /

pūrvaṃ yaḥ kathito'bhyāsaścaturdhā taṃ parityajet /83/

divā vā yadi vā rātrau yāmamātraṃ samabhyaset /

eka bāraṃ pratidinaṃ kuryāt kevalakumbhakam /84/

[34]

Then, there appear signs (in this stage in the body of the yogi). I will describe some of them. The previously mentioned practice of *kumbhaka* four times a day should be given up. The *kevala kumbhaka* alone should be practiced properly for three hours either during the day or at night everyday. -83-84.

Perfect Kumbhaka Is Pratyāhāra

प्रत्याहारो हि एवं स्यादेवं कर्त्तुर्हि योगिनः ।

इन्द्रियाणीन्द्रियार्थेभ्यो यत्प्रत्याहरति स्फुटम् ।

योगी कुम्भकमास्थाय प्रत्याहारः स उच्यते ॥८५॥

pratyāhāro hi evaṃ syādevaṃ karturhi yoginaḥ /

indriyāṇīndriyārthebhyo yatpratyāharati sphuṭam /

yogī kumbhakamāsthāya pratyāhāraḥ sa ucyate /85/

Pratyāhāra will certainly begin to arise in the yogi by practicing in this way. When the senses are withdrawn from their respective sense-organs and their objects completely and the yogi is established in *kumbhaka*, it is called *pratyāhāra*. -85.

Pratyāhāra Practice

यद्यत्पश्यति चक्षुर्भ्यां तत्तदात्मनि भावयेत् ।

यद्यज्जिघ्रति नासाभ्यां तत्तदात्मनि भावयेत् ।

जिह्वया यद्रसयति तत्तदात्मनि भावयेत् ।

त्वचा यद्यत्सम्स्पृशति तत्तदात्मनि भावयेत् ॥८७॥

yadyatpaśyati cakṣurbhyāṃ tattadātmani bhāvayet /

yadyajjighrati nāsābhyāṃ tattadātmani bhāvayet /

jihvayā yadrasayati tattadātmani bhāvayet /

tvacā yadyatsamspriti tattadātmani bhaavayet /87/

While practicing *pratyāhāra*, whatever the yogi sees through his eyes, smells through his nostrils, tastes through his tongue and touches through his skins (i.e. the five sense organs), he should feel that it is the *Ātman* (the Self). -87.

एवं ज्ञानेन्द्रियाणां हि तत्संख्यावस्तु सन्धयेत् ।

याममात्रं प्रतिदिनं योगी यत्नादतन्द्रितः ॥८८॥

evaṃ jñānendriyāṇāṃ hi tatsaṅkhyāvastu sandhayet /

yāmamātraṃ pratidinaṃ yogī yatnādatandritaḥ /88/

In this way, the yogi should carefully withdraw himself from his senses and their respective organs and unite (with *Ātman*) without any tiredness for three hours everyday. -88.

Pratyāhāra Practice Bestows Siddhis

तदा विचित्रसामर्थ्यं योगिनां जायते धुवम् ।

दूरशुतिः दूरदृष्टिः क्षणाद्दूरगमस्तथा ॥८९॥

वाक्सिद्धिः कामचारित्वमदृश्यकरणं तथा ।

मलमूत्रप्रलेपेन लोहादीनां सुवर्णता ।

खेचरत्वं तथान्यत्तु सतताभ्यासयोगिनः ॥९०॥

tadā vicitrasāmarthyaṃ yogināṃ jāyate dhruvam /

[36]

dūraśrutiḥ dūradṛṣṭiḥ kṣaṇāddūragamastathā /89/

vāksiddhiḥ kāmacāritvamadṛśyakaraṇaṃ tathā /

malamūtrapralepena lohādīnāṃ suvarṇatā /

khecaratvaṃ tathānyattu satatābhyāsayoginaḥ /90/

As a result (of the practice of *pratyāhāra*), there arise miraculous powers in the yogi: clairaudience, clairvoyance, ability to reach anywhere instantly, supernatural perfection in speech, power to do anything and power to be invisible at his will, power to converting iron and other metals into gold by rubbing them with his faeces and urine and the power of moving into the space and other (supernatural) powers through his constant practice. -89-90.

Siddhis Obstacles to Mahāsiddhi

तदा बुद्धिमता भाव्यं योगिना योगसिद्धये ।

एते विघ्नाः महासिद्धेर्न रमेत्तेषु बुद्धिमान् ॥९१॥

tadā buddhimatā bhāvyaṃ yoginā yogasiddhaye /

ete vighnāḥ mahāsiddherna rametteṣu buddhimān /91/

Then the wise yogi in order to gain perfection in yoga should consider that these (supernatural powers) are obstacles to *mahāsiddhi* (great perfection) and should not rejoice in them at all. -91.

No Demonstration of Powers

न दर्शयेच्च कस्मैचित् स्वसामर्थ्य हि सर्वदा ।

कदाचिद् दर्शयेत्प्रीत्या भक्तियुक्ताय वा पुनः ॥९२॥

यथा मूर्खो यथा मूढो यथा बधिर एव वा ।

तथा वर्तेत लोकेषु स्वसामर्थ्यस्य गुप्तये ॥९३॥

na darśayecca kasmaicit svasāmarthya hi sarvadā /

kadācid darśayetprītyā bhaktiyuktāya vā punaḥ /92/

yathā mūrkho yathā mūḍho yathā badhira eva vā /

tathā varteta lokeṣu svasāmarthyasya guptaye /93/

The yogi should never demonstrate his powers to anyone. He may show them due to his love to the one who is established in devotion. He should remain in public as though he were a fool, an ignorant or a deaf so that he can keep his powers secret. -92-93.

Focus on Practice Alone

नोचेच्छिष्याः हि बहवो भवन्त्येव न संशयः ।

तत्कर्मकरणव्यग्रः स्वाभ्यासे विस्मृतो भवेत् ।

अभ्यासेन विहीनस्तु ततो लौकिकतां व्रजेत् ॥९४॥

nocecchiṣyāḥ hi bahavo bhavanti sva na saṃśayaḥ /

tatkarmakaraṇavyagraḥ svābhyāse vismṛto bhavet /

abhyāsena vihīnastu tato laukikatāṃ vrajet /94/

Else, he will have many disciples withour any doubt. He will be occupied by their work and will be forgetful about his own practice. Without yoga practice, he becomes/remains like a public person in general. -94.

Ghaṭāvasthā through Constant Practice

अविस्मृत्य गुरोर्वाक्यमभ्यसेत्तदहर्निशम् ।

एवं भवेद् घटावस्था सदाभ्यासस्य योगिनः ॥९५॥

avismṛtya gurorvakyamabhyasettadaharniśam /

evaṃ bhaved ghaṭāvasthā sadābhyāsasya yoginaḥ /95/

Without forgetting the words of his guru, he should contstantly practice day and night. In this way, the yogi attains *ghaṭāvasthā* (the pot or vessel stage) through his regular practice. -95.

Discussion and Meeting Worthless

अनभ्यासेन योगस्य वृथा गोष्ठ्या न सिध्यति ।

तस्मात् सर्वप्रयत्नेन योगमेव सदाभ्यसेत् ॥९६॥

anabhyāsena yogasya vṛthā goṣṭhyā na sidhyati /

tasmāt sarvaprayatnena yogameva sadābhyaset /96/

One cannot attain perfection in yoga without practice and involving oneslf in worthless discussion and meeting. Therefore, the yogi should constantly practice yoga with all efforts. -96.

The Kuṇḍalīnī Awakens In Paricayāvasthā

ततः परिचयावस्था जायतेऽभ्यासयोगतः ।

वायुः सम्प्रेरितो यत्नाद् अग्निना सह कुण्डलीम् ॥९७॥

बोधयित्वा सुषुम्रायां प्रविशेदविरोधतः ।

वायुना सह चित्तन्तु प्रविशेच्च महापथम् ॥९८॥

tataḥ paricayāvasthā jāyate'abhyāsayogataḥ /

vāyuḥ samprerito yatnād agninā saha kuṇḍalīm /97/

bodhayitvā suṣumnāyāṃ praviśedavirodhataḥ /

vāyunā saha cittantu praviśecca mahāpatham /98/

Then *paricayāvasthā* occurs for a yogi through the continuous practice of yoga. The *vāyu* driven by the fire awakens the *kuṇḍalīnī* and it enters into the *suṣumnā* without any obstruction. The *chitta* also enters into *mahāpatha* (literally, the great path) along with the *vāyu*. -97-98.

महापथं श्मशानं च सुषुम्राप्येकमेव हि ।

नाम्रां मतान्तरे भेदः फले भेदो न विद्यते ॥९९॥

mahāpathaṃ śmaśānaṃ ca suṣumnāpyekameva hi /

nāmnāṃ matāntare bhedaḥ phale bhedo na vidyate /99/

Mahāpatha (the great path), *śmaśāna* (the burial ground) and *suṣumnā* are certainly synonymous and the same. There are different opinions for for different names, but the difference does not exist in the result. -99.

Knowledge of the Present, Future and Past

वर्तमानं भविष्यञ्च भूतार्थं चापि वेत्यसौ ।

यस्य चित्तं सपवनं सुषुम्रां प्रविशेदिह ॥१००॥

vartamānaṃ bhaviṣyañca bhūtārthaṃ cāpi vetyasau /

yasya cittaṃ sapavanaṃ suṣumnāṃ praviśediha /100/

The yogi whose *chitta* enters into *suṣumnā* along with the *pavana* (the air or *vāyu*) knows the present, future and past at once. -100.

Practice of Five Dhāraṇas on Five Bhūtas

भाव्यानर्थान् स विज्ञाय योगि रहसि यत्नतः ।

पञ्चधा धारणं कुर्यात् तत्तद्भूतभयापहम् ॥१०१॥

bhāvyānarthān saḥ vijñāya yogi rahasi yatnataḥ /

pañcadhā dhāraṇam kuryāt tattadbhūtabhayāpaham /101/

Having known the events that occur in the future, the yogi effortfully should remain in an isolated place and then practice the five types of *dhāraṇas* (concentrations) in order to remove the fears of five *bhūtas* (elements) respectively. -101.

Practice of Prithivi Dhāraṇā

पृथिवीधारणं वक्ष्ये पार्थिवेभ्यो भयापहम् ।

नाभेरधो गुदस्योर्ध घटिकाः पञ्च धारयेत् ॥१०२॥

वायुं भवेत्ततो पृथ्वीधारणं तद्भयापहम् ।

पृथिवीसम्भवस्तस्य न मृत्युर्योगिनो भवेत् ॥१०३॥

pṛthivīdhāraṇam vakṣye pārthivebhyo bhayāpaham /

nābheradho gudasyordhvam ghaṭikāḥ pañca dhārayet /102/

vāyum bhavet tato pṛthvīdhāraṇam tadbhayāpaham /

pṛthivīsambhavastasya na mṛtyuryogino bhavet /103/

Now I am going to tell you about the *prithvi dhāraṇā* (concentration on earth element) in order to destroy the fear of the objects that arise from the earth. For the practice of this *dhāraṇā* the yogi should retain his prana under the navel and above the anus for five *ghatis* (two hours). This practice is called *prithvi dhāraṇā* which removes all the obstacles/fears that arise through worldly objects.

There is no possibility of death of the yogi due to the objects related to earth element. – 102-103.

Practice of Jala Dhāraṇā

नाभिस्थाने ततो वायुं धारयेत्पञ्चनाडिकाः ।

ततो जलाद् भयं नास्ति जलमृत्युर्न योगिनः ॥१०४॥

nābhisthāne tato vāyuṃ dhārayetpañcanāḍikāḥ /

tato jalād bhayaṃ nāsti jalamṛtyurna yoginaḥ /104/

Through the retention of *prāṇa* for five *ghatis* at the navel area, there will be no fear of water. The yogi will not face his death due to water or water element. -104.

Practice of Āgneyi Dhāraṇā

नाभ्युर्ध्वमण्डले वायुं धारयेत्पञ्चनाडिकाः ।

आग्नेयधारणा सेयं न मृत्युर्तस्य वह्निना ॥१०५॥

nābhyurdhvamaṇḍale vāyuṃ dhārayetpañcanāḍikāḥ /

agneyadhāraṇā seyaṃ na mṛtyurtasya vahninā /105/

The yogi should retain the *vāyu* for five *ghatis* on the sphere above the navel. It is *āgneyi dhāraṇā*. The fire cannot kill him (by the practice of this *dhāraṇā*). -104.

सदा विचित्रसामर्थ्यं योगिनो जायते ध्रुवम् ।

न दह्यते शरीरं च प्रक्षिप्तो वह्निकुण्डके ॥१०५॥

sadā vicitrasāmarthyaṃ yogino jāyate dhruvam /

na dahyate śarīraṃ ca prakṣipto vahnikuṇḍake /105/

The yogi indeed ever attains amazing power. Even if his body is thrown into the *vahni/agni kuṇḍa* (a round hole of the flaming fire in the ground), it is not burned. -105.

Practice of Vāyu Dhāraṇā

वक्षभ्रुवोहि मध्ये तु प्रदेशत्रयसंयुते ।

धारयेत्पञ्चघटिकाः वायुं सैषा हि वायवी ।

धारणात्तत्र वायोस्तु योगिनो न भयं भवेत् ॥१०६॥

vakshabhruvohi madhye tu pradeśatrayasaṃyute /

dhārayetpañcaghaṭikāḥ vāyuṃ saiṣā hi vāyavī /

dhāraṇāttatra vāyostu yogino na bhayaṃ bhavet /106/

The yogi should hold the *vāyu* for five *ghatis* by combining the three regions - *anāhata*, *vishuddha* and *ājna* located between the *vaksha* (chest) and the *bhrumadhya* (eyebrow center). This is *vāyavī dhāraṇā*. By the practice of *vāyu dhāraṇā* there, the yogi will not have the fear of the *vāyu*. -106.

Practice of Ākāśa Dhāraṇā

भूमध्यादुपरिष्टात्तु धारयेत्पञ्चनाडिकाः ।

वायुं योगी प्रयत्नेन सेयमाकाशधारणा ॥१०७॥

आकाशधारणां कुर्वन्मृत्युं जयति तत्त्वतः ।

यत्र तत्र स्थितो वापि सुखमत्यन्तमश्रुते ॥१०८॥

bhrūmadhyādupariṣṭāttu dhārayetpañcanāḍikāḥ /

vāyuṃ yogī prayatnena seyamākāśadhāraṇā /107/

ākāśadhāraṇāṃ kurvanmṛtyuṃ jayati tattvataḥ /

yatra tatra sthito vāpi sukhamatyantamaśnute /108/

When the yogi retains the *prāṇa vāyu* with due effort for two hours above the eyebrow center, this is called *ākāśa dhāraṇā*. The yogi who practices *ākāśa dhāraṇā* defeats the death in reality. Wherever he lives, he enjoys supreme happiness. -107-108.

Practice of Five Dhāraṇās Defeat Death

एवं च धारणाः पञ्च कुर्याद्योगी विचक्षणः ।

ततो दृढशरीरः स्यात्मृत्युर्तस्य न विद्यते ॥१०९॥

इत्येवं पञ्चभूतानां धारणां यः समभ्यसेत् ।

ब्रह्मणः प्रलये वापि मृत्युर्तस्य न विद्यते ॥११०॥

evaṃ ca dhāraṇāḥ pañca kuryādyogī vicakṣaṇaḥ /

tato dṛḍhaśarīraḥ syanmṛtyurtasya na vidyate /109/

ityevaṃ pañcabhūtānāṃ dhāraṇāṃ yaḥ samabhyaset /

brahmaṇaḥ pralaye vāpi mṛtyurtasya na vidyate /110/

In this way, the wise yogi should practice the five *dhāraṇās*. Then his body becomes robust and death does not exist for him. One who properly practices these five *dhāraṇās* on the five elements in this way, he will not face death even at the time of *brahma pralaya* (the dissolution of the whole world). -109-110.

Meditation on Iṣṭadevatā after Pañcadhāraṇā Practice

समभ्यसेत्तदा ध्यानं घटिकाः षष्टिमेव च ।

वायुं निरुद्ध्य ध्यायेत्तु देवतामिष्टदायिनीम् ॥१११॥

samabhyasettadā dhyānaṃ ghaṭikāḥ ṣaṣṭimeva ca /

vāyuṃ niruddhya dhyāyettu devatāmiṣṭadāyinīm /111/

Then the yogi should duly practice *dhyāna* for 24 hours. By holding his *prāṇa vāyu*, he should meditate on his *devatā* (favourable deity) *iṣṭadāyinī* (who fulfills one's desires). -111.

Saguṇa Dhyāna Bestows Siddhis, Nirguṇa Liberation

सगुणध्यानमेवं स्यादणिमादिगुणप्रदम् ।

निर्गुणं खमिव ध्यात्वा मोक्षमार्गं प्रपद्यते ॥११२॥

saguṇadhyānamevaṃ syādaṇimādiguṇapradam /

nirguṇaṃ khamiva dhyātvā mokṣamārgaṃ prapadyate /112/

Saguṇa dhyāna (meditation on the form of God or deity with attributes) thus bestows the power of *aṇimā*, etc., *siddhis* (supernatural powers). By meditating on the attributeless space (the *nirguṇa* form of *brahman*), one arrives at *mokṣa mārga* (the path of liberation). -112.

Practice of Samādhi after Nirguṇa Dhyāna

निर्गुणध्यानसम्पन्नः समाधिं च ततोऽभ्यसेत् ।

दिनद्वादशकेनैव समाधिं समवाप्नुयात् ॥११३॥

वायुं निरुध्य मेधावी जीवन्मुक्तो भवेद् ध्रुवम् ।

समाधिः समताऽवस्था जीवात्मपरमात्मनोः ॥११४॥

nirguṇadhyānasampannaḥ samādhiṃ ca tato'bhyaset /

dinadvādaśakenaiva samādhiṃ samavāpnuyāt /113/

vāyuṃ nirudhya medhāvī jīvanmukto bhaved dhruvam /

samādhiḥ samatā'vasthā jīvātmaparamātmanoḥ /114/

Having well established in *nirguṇa dhyāna* (on the formless form of *Brahman*), then the yogi should practice for the realization of *samādhi*. He can duly attain *samādhi* within twelve days. Having controlled his *vāyu*, the wise yogi certainly attains liberation from life. *Samadhi* is identical stage between *jīvātmā* (the Individual Self) and *paramātmā* (the Supreme Self). -113-114.

Dissolution after Discarding All Types of Karmas

यदि स्याद् देहमुत्स्रष्टुमिच्छा तदुत्सृजेत्स्वयम् ।

परब्रह्मणि लीयेत त्यक्त्वा कर्मशुभाशुभम् ॥११५॥

अथ चेन्नो समुत्स्रष्टुं स्वशरीरं यदि प्रियम् ।

सर्व लोकेषु विचरेदणिमादिगुणान्वितः ॥११६॥

yadi syād dehamutsraṣṭumicchā tadutsṛjetsvayam /

parabrahmaṇi līyeta tyaktvā karmaśubhāśubham /115/

atha cenno samutsraṣṭuṃ svaśarīraṃ yadi priyam /

sarva lokeṣu vicaredaṇimādiguṇānvitaḥ /116/

If the yogi wants to give up his body, he can do so himself (as per his wish). Then, having abandoned all types of good or bad karmas, he should dissolve (his Individual Self) into the Supreme Self. Furthermore, if his body is dear to him and does not want to give it up, then he should roam over the whole world with supernatural powers like *aṇimā* and others. -115-116.

The Yogi Leading a life as Maheśvara

कदाचित्स्वेच्छया देवो भूत्वा स्वर्गेऽपि संचरेत् ।

मनुष्यो वापि यक्षो वा स्वेच्छया हि क्षणाद् भवेत् ॥११७॥

सिंहो व्याघ्रो गजो वा स्यादिच्छया जन्तुतां व्रजेत् ।

यथेष्टमेव वर्त्तेत योगी विद्वान्महेश्वरः ॥११८॥

kadācitsvecchayā devo bhūtvā svarge'pi saṃcaret /

manuṣyo vāpi yakṣo vā svecchayā hi kṣaṇād bhavet /117/

siṃho vyāghro gajo vā syādicchayā jantutāṃ vrajet /

yatheṣṭameva vartteta yogī vidvānmaheśvaraḥ /118/

He may become a divine being if he wish so and go to heaven. He may change himself into a man or a *yakṣa* (a type of demi-god) in no time. He can become an aminal as he wishes – a lion, a tiger, an elephant or a horse. Thus the wise yogi follows his course of life at his will as *Maheśvara*. -117-118.

Aṣṭāṅgayoga – The Path of Kavimārga

कविमार्गोऽयमुक्तस्ते साङ्कृते अष्टाङ्गयोगतः ।

सिद्धानां कपिलादीनां मतं वक्ष्ये ततः परम् ।

अभ्यासभेदतो भेदः फलं तु सममेव हि ॥११९॥

kavimārgo'yamuktaste sāṅkṛte aṣṭāṅgayogataḥ /

siddhānāṃ kapilādīnāṃ mataṃ vakṣye tataḥ param /

abhyāsabhedato bhedaḥ phalaṃ tu samameva hi /119/

O *Sāṅkṛti*! I have told you the *aṣṭāṅgayoga* (the yoga of eight parts or limbs) according to *kavimārga* (the way it was taught by the ancient sages). Now I am going to tell you the opinions of the *siddhas* like sage *Kapila* and others (on yoga). The difference is there in the way of practice (of the two); but the result (of both) is surely the same. - 119.

Mahāmudrā Practice

महामुद्रां प्रवक्ष्यामि भैरवेणोक्तमादरात् ।

पार्ष्णिवामस्य पादस्य योनिस्थाने नियोजयेत् ॥१२०॥

प्रसार्य दक्षिणं पादं हस्ताभ्यां धारयेद् दृढम् ।

चिबुकं हृदि विन्यस्य पूरयेत् वायुना पुनः ॥१२१॥

कुम्भकेन यथाशक्त्या धारयित्वा तु रेचयेत् ।

वामाङ्गेन समभ्यस्य दक्षिणाङ्गेन चाभ्यसेत् ॥१२२॥

mahāmudrāṃ pravakṣyāmi bhairaveṇoktamādarāt /

pārṣṇivāmasya pādasya yonisthāne niyojayet /120/

prasārya dakṣiṇaṃ pādaṃ hastābhyāṃ dhārayed dṛḍham /

cibukaṃ hṛdi vinyasya pūrayet vāyunā punaḥ /121/

kumbhakena yathāśaktyā dhārayitvā tu recayet /

vāmāṅgena samabhyasya dakṣiṇāṅgena cābhyaset /122/

Now I will describe *mahāmudrā* as taught by *Bhairava* with great respect. The heel of the left foot should be placed against the perineum extending the right foot. It should be held firmly with both hands. Having placed the chin on the heart (chest), one should fill up with the air. *Kumbhaka* should be performed for as long as possible and then the air should be exhaled. After properly practicing it with the left leg, it should also be practiced with the right leg. -120-122.

Mahābandha Practice

प्रसारितस्तु यः पादस्तमूरूपरि विन्यसेत् ।

अयमेव महाबन्धो मुद्रावच्चामुमभ्यसेत् ॥१२३॥

prasāritastu yaḥ pādastamurūpari vinyaset /

ayameva mahābandho mudrāvaccāmumabhyaset /123/

This is called *mahābandha* when the extended foot is kept on the thigh (of the opposite leg). It should also be practiced similar to *Mahāmudrā*. -123.

महाबन्धस्थितो भूमौ स्फिचौ सन्ताडयेच्छनै: ।

अयमेव महाबन्ध: सिद्धै: अभ्यस्यते नरै: ॥१२४॥

mahābandhasthito bhūmau sphicau santāḍayecchanaiḥ /

ayameva mahābandhaḥ siddhaiḥ abhyasyate naraiḥ /124/

The yogi seated in the *mahābandha* should gently strike on the ground with his buttocks. This *mahābandha* is practiced by perfected noblemen. -124.

Khecarī Mudra Practice

अन्त: कपालकुहरे जिह्वां व्यावर्त्य बन्धयेत् ।

भूमध्ये दृष्टिरप्येषा मुद्रा भवति खेचरी ॥१२५॥

antaḥ kapālakuhare jihvāṃ vyāvartya bandhayet /

bhrūmadhye dṛṣṭirapyeṣā mudrā bhavati khecarī /125/

The tongue should be turned back and held into the cavity of the skull and the vision should be focused on the eyebrow center. This is in called *khecarī mudrā.* -126.

Jālandhara Bandha Practice

कण्ठमाकुञ्च्य हृदये स्थापयेद् दृढमिच्छया ।

जलन्धरो बन्ध एषो ह्यमृतद्रवपालकः ॥१२६॥

kaṇṭhamākuñcya hṛdaye sthāpayed dṛḍhamicchayā /

jālandharo bandha eṣa amṛtadravapālakaḥ /126/

The chin should ben contracted and placed on the chest with the firm willpower. This is called *jālandhara bandha.* This *bandha* is the protector of *amṛta drava* (the immortal liquid). -126.

नाभिस्थोऽग्निः कपालस्थसहस्रकमलच्युतम् ।

अमृतं सर्वदा तावद् अन्तर्ज्वलति देहिनाम् ॥१२७॥

nābhistho'gniḥ kapālasthasahasrakamalacyutam /

amṛtaṃ sarvadā tāvad antarjvalati dehinām /127/

The fire situated at the navel always burns internally so long as the *amṛta* is dripping from the thousand-pettalled lotus in the skull of all human beings. -127.

Drinking of the Amṛta Oneself

यथा चाग्निस्तदमृतं न पिबेत्तु पिबेत्स्वयम् ।

याति पश्चिममार्गेण एवमभ्यासतः सदा ।

अमृतं कुरुते देहं जालन्धरमतोऽभ्यसेत् ॥१२८॥

yathā cāgnistadamṛtaṃ na pibettu pibetsvayam /

yāti paścimamārgeṇa evamabhyāsataḥ sadā /

amṛtaṃ kurute dehaṃ jalandharamato 'bhyaset /128/

The yogi should drink the *amṛta* himself so that the fire (at the navel) may not drink or burn it. Through regular practice in this way, it goes through the reverse path and it makes the body immortal. Therefore, one should practice *jālandhara bandha.* -128.

Uddiyāna Bandha Practice

उड्याणं तु सहजं गुणौघात् कथितं सदा ।

अभ्यसेदस्ततन्द्रस्तु वृद्धोऽपि तरुणो भवेत् ॥१२९॥

नाभेः ऊर्ध्वमधश्चापि तानं कुर्यात्प्रयत्न तः ।

षण्मासमभ्यसेन्मृत्युं जयेदेव न संशयः ॥१३०॥

uḍyānaṃ tu sahajaṃ guṇaughāt kathitaṃ sadā /

abhyasedastatandrastu vṛddho 'pi taruṇo bhavet /129/

nābheḥ ūrdhvamadhaścāpi tānaṃ kuryātprayatnataḥ /

ṣaṇmāsamabhyasenmṛtyuṃ jayedeva na saṃśayaḥ /130/

It is said that the *uddiyāna bandha* is always *sahaja* (natural/easy to practice) and *guṇaughāt* (due to its qualities of destroying diseases and aging). When it is practiced regularly withour laziness, even a man in old age would become a young man. With due effort the abdomen above and below the navel area should be drawn upward. When it is practiced for six months, death is surely conquered without doubt. -129-130.

Mūla Bandha Practice

मूलबन्धं तु यो नित्यमभ्यसेत्स च योगवित् ।

गुदे पार्ष्णिं तु सम्पीड्य वायुमाकुञ्चयेद् बलात् ।

वारं वारं यथा चोर्ध्वं समायाति समीरणः ॥१३१॥

mūlabandhaṃ tu yo nityamabhyasetsa ca yogavit /

gude pārṣṇiṃ tu sampīḍya vāyumākuñcayed balāt /

vāraṃ vāraṃ yathā cordhvaṃ samāyāti samīraṇaḥ /131/

One who regularly practices *mūla bandha* is the knower of yoga. One should press his anus with his heel and contract the perineum with force. It should be reapeted again and again in order to force the *samīra* (*apāna vāyu*) move upward. -131.

Union of Prāṇa and Apāna, Nāda and Bindū

प्राणापानौ नादबिन्दू मूलबन्धेन चैकताम् ।

गत्वा योगस्य संसिद्धिं यच्छतो नात्र संशयः ॥१३२॥

prāṇāpānau nādabindū mūlabandhena caikatām /

gatvā yogasya saṃsiddhiṃ yacchato nātra saṃśayaḥ /132/

Prāṇa and *apāna*, *nāda* and *bindū* are united through *mūla bandha*. When this union takes place, it grants complete accomplishment in yoga without any doubt. -132.

Viparita Karaṇa Practice

करणं विपरिताख्यं सर्वव्याधिविनाशनम् ।

नित्यमभ्यासयुक्तस्य जठराग्निः विवर्द्धते ॥१३३॥

आहारो बहुलः तस्य सम्पाद्यः साङ्कृते ध्रुवम् ।

अल्पाहारो यदि भवेदग्निः दाहं करोति वै ।

ऊर्ध्वं भानुरधश्चन्द्रस्तद्यथा शृणु साङ्कृते ॥१३४॥

karaṇam viparitākhyaṃ sarvavyādhivināśanam /

nityamabhyāsayuktasya jaṭharāgniḥ vivarddhate /133 /

āhāro bahulaḥ tasya sampādyaḥ sāṅkṛte dhruvam

alpāhāro yadi bhavedagniḥ dāhaṃ karoti vai /

ūrdhvaṃ bhānuradhaścandrastadyathā śṛṇu sāṅkṛte /134/

The *mudrā* called *viparita karaṇa* destroys all types of diseases. One who regularly practices it, his digestive fire will be increased. Therefore, O *Sāṅkṛti*! Provision of sufficient food should be made for him. If there will not be sufficient food, his body will surely be consumed by the digestive fire. Now listen, O *Sāṅkṛti*! I tell you how the sun goes up and the moon goes down. -133-134.

अधः शिरश्चोर्ध्वपादः क्षणं स्यात्प्रथमे दिने ।

क्षणात्तु किंचिदधिकमभ्यसेन दिने दिने ॥१३५॥

वलिश्च पलितश्चैव षण्मासोर्ध्वं न दृश्यते ।

याममात्रं तु यो नित्यमभ्यसेत्स तु योगवित् ॥१३६॥

adhaḥ śiraścordhvapādaḥ kṣaṇaṃ syātprathame dine /

kṣaṇāttu kimcidadhikamabhyasena dine dine /135/

valiśca palitaścaiva ṣaṇmāsordhvaṃ na dṛśyate /

yāmamātraṃ tu yo nityamabhyasetsa tu ogavit /136/

The head should be up and and the feet down for a short time on the very first day. Then the duration of its practice should be increased a little bit more daily. By practicing it regularly after six months grey hairs and wrinkles will not be seen. One who practices it for three hours daily he will become the knower of yoga. -135-136.

Vajroli Practice

वज्रोलिं कथयिष्यामि गोपितं सर्वयोगिभिः ।

अतीवैतद् रहस्यं हि न देयं यस्य कस्यचित् ।

स्वप्राणैस्तु समो यो स्यात्तस्मै च कथयेद् धुवम् ॥१३७॥

vajroliṃ kathayiṣyāmi gopitaṃ sarvayogibhiḥ /

atīvaitad rahasyaṃ hi na deyaṃ yasya kasyacit /

svaprāṇaistu samo yo syāttasamai ca kathayed dhruvam /137/

Now I will explain you the *vajroli* which is kept secret by all yogis. For it is top-secret, so it should not be given to everyone. It should be surely imparted to him who is equal to one's own *prāṇa* (the soul of the giver himself). -137.

स्वेच्छया वर्त्तमानोऽपि योगोक्तनियमैर्विना ।

वज्रोलिं यो विजानाति स योगी सिद्धिभाजनः ॥१३८॥

svecchayā varttamāno'pi yogoktaniyamairvinā /

vajroliṃ yo vijānati sa yogī siddhibhājanaḥ /138/

The yogi who knows *vajroli* is entitled to perfection in yoga even if he does not follow the specified rules in yoga and also leads his life according to his will. -138.

Two Rare Things for Vajroli Practice

तत्र वस्तु द्वयं वक्ष्ये दुर्लभं येन केनचित् ।

लभ्यते यदि तस्यैव योगसिद्धिकरं स्मृतम् ॥१३९॥

tatra vastu dvayaṃ vakṣye durlabhaṃ yena kenacit /

labhyate yadi tasyaiva yogasiddhikaraṃ smṛtam /139/

There are two things, I am telling you, which are rare to find for anyone. If those two are available, it is considered that they grant perfection in yoga. -139.

Aṅgirasa Is the Rarest

क्षीरमाङ्गिरसं चेति द्वयोराद्यं तु लभ्यते ।

द्वितीयं दुर्लभं पुंसां स्त्रीभ्यः साध्यमुपायतः ।

योगाभ्यासरता स्त्री च पुंसां यत्नेतः साधयेत् ॥१४०॥

kṣīramāṅgirasaṃ ceti dvayorādyaṃ tu labhyate /

dvitīyaṃ durlabhaṃ puṃsāṃ strībhyaḥ sādhyamupāyataḥ /

yogābhyāsaratā strī ca puṃsāṃ yatnena sādhayet /140/

These are *kṣīra* (milk) and *aṅgirasa* (the seminal fluid). Of these two, the first is (easily) available, but the second one is very rare. The yogis should obtain it from women by some means. A yogi, by efforts, should accomplish it with a yogini who is devoted to the practice of yoga. -140.

No Concern of Gender in Vajroli Practice

पुमान् स्त्री वा यदन्योऽन्यं स्त्रीपुंस्त्वानपेक्षया ।

स्वप्रयोजनमात्रैकसाधनात्सिद्धिमाप्नुयात् ॥१४१॥

pumān strī vā yadanyonyaṃ strīpuṃstvānapekṣayā /

svaprayojanamātraikasādhanātsiddhimāpnuyāt /141/

When a yogi or yogini has or both of them have no concern at all with his/her or their gender or when the feeling/emotion toward one another between the two male and female *vajroli* partners is above the level of sexual concern and practice only for attaining his/her or their goal will achieve *siddhis* (perfections) through the practice of *vajroli*. -141.

Drawing Back Bindu for Preservation

चलितो यदि बिन्दुस्तमुर्ध्वमाकृष्य रक्षयेत् ।

एवं च रक्षितो बिन्दुः मृत्युं जयति तत्त्वतः ॥१४२॥

calito yadi bindustamurdhvamākṛṣya rakṣayet /

evaṃ ca rakṣito binduḥ mṛtuṃ jayati tattvataḥ /142/

If *bindu* (the seminal fluid) moves out (during the practice of *vajroli*), one should draw it upward (for taking it back) and preserve it. If *bindu* is preserved in this way, one truly gains victory over death. -142.

Life Depends on Bindu

मरणं बिन्दुपातेन जीवनं बिन्दुधारणात् ।

बिन्दुरक्षाप्रसादेन सर्वं सिध्यति योगिनः ॥१४३॥

maraṇaṃ bindupātena jīvanaṃ bindudhāraṇat /

bindurakṣāprasādena sarvaṃ sidhyati yoginaḥ /143/

Death occurs by the loss of *bindu*, life exists/remains by the preservation of *bindu*. By the gift of *bindu* protection, the yogis achieve all perfections. -143.

Practice of Amaroli and Sahajoli

अमरोलिस्तद्यथा स्यात्सहजोलिस्ततो यथा ।

तदभ्यासक्रमः शस्यः सिद्धानां सम्प्रदायतः ॥१४४॥

amarolistadyathā syātsahajolistato yathā /

tadabhyāsakramaḥ śasyaḥ siddhānāṃ sampradāyataḥ /144/

The *amaroli* and *sahajoli* are similar practices and modifications of the same practice. The order and method of their practice are followed according to the tradition of *siddhas*. -144.

Rājayoga Occurs by Practice as Time Passes

एतैः सर्वैस्तु कथितैरभ्यसेत् कालकालतः ।

ततो भवेद् राजयोगो नान्तरा भवति ध्रुवम् ।

न दिङ्मात्रेण सिद्धिरस्यादभ्यसेनैव जायते ॥१४५॥

etaiḥ sarvaistu kathitairabhyaset kālakālataḥ /

tato bhaved rājayogo nāntarā bhavati dhruvam /

na dinmātreṇa siddhissyādabhyasenaiva jāyate /145/

All those aforesaid methods of practices should be performed in due course of time. Then *rājayoga* will occur; otherwise, it will not.

Perfection can be accomplished through constant practice, but not by mere (theoretical) learning. -145.

A Real Rājayogi Acts as Per His Desire

राजयोगं वरं प्राप्य सर्वसत्त्ववशङ्करम् ।

सर्वं कुर्यान्न वा कुर्याद् यथारुचिविचेष्टितम् ॥१४६॥

rājayogaṃ varaṃ prāpya sarvasattvavaśaṅkaram /

sarvaṃ kuryānna vā kuryād yathāruciviceṣṭitam /146/

After getting the boon of *rājayoga*, the yogi gains power to control all creatures. He can do everything or nothing and can act as per his desire. -146.

Completion of Internal Kriyā Results in Niṣpatti

यथान्तरा च योगेन निष्पन्ना योगिनः क्रिया ।

यथावस्था हि निष्पत्तिर्भुक्तिमुक्तिफलप्रदा ॥१४७॥

yathāntarā ca yogena niṣpannā yoginaḥ kriyā /

yathāvasthā hi niṣpattirbhuktimuktiphalapradā /147/

When the *kriyā* of internal yoga of a yogi is complete, that is certainly the stage of *niṣpatti* (the completion of highest perfection in yoga), which grants the fruits of *bhukti* (enjoyment) and *mukti* (liberation). -147.

Completion of Discourse, Achievement of Siddhis

सर्वं ते कथितं ब्रह्मन् सांस्कृते योगमाचर ।

इति तस्य वचः शुत्वा सांस्कृतियोगमाप्नवान् ।

[58]

सर्वासिद्धीमवाप्यासौ दत्तात्रेयप्रसादतः ॥१४८॥

sarvaṃ te kathitaṃ brahman sāṅskṛte yogamācara /

iti tasya vacaḥ śrutvā Sāṅkṛtiḥ yogamāptavān /

sarvāsiddhīmavāpyāsau dattātreyaprasādataḥ /148/

O *Brahman*! I have explained you everything. O *Sāṅkṛti*! Now you should practice yoga. After hearing those words of *Dattātreya*, *Sāṅkṛti* acquired yogic perfection and all the *siddhis* through the blessing of *Dattātreya*. -148.

Gradual Perfection through Sādhanā

य इदं पठते नित्यं साधुभ्यः श्रावयेदपि ।

तस्य योगः क्रमेणैव सिध्यत्येव न संशयः ॥१४९॥

ya idaṃ paṭhate nityaṃ sādhubhyaḥ śrāvayedapi /

tasya yogaḥ krameṇaiva sidhyatyeva na saṃśayaḥ /149/

One who regularly reads it or makes *sādhus* (noblemen) listen it will attain gradual perfection in yoga without any doubt. -149.

Freedom from Death by Devoted Practice

योगिनोऽभ्यासयुक्ताः ये ह्यरण्येषु गृहेषु वा ।

बहुकालं रमन्ते स्म बहुकालविवर्जिताः ॥१५०॥

yogino'bhyāsayuktāḥ ye hyaraṇyeṣu gṛheṣu vā /

bahukālaṃ ramante sma bahukālavivarjitāḥ /150/

Those yogis who are devoted to practice whether living in the forest or at home enjoy for a long time being free from many recurring deaths. -150.

Futile Life without Yoga Practice

तस्मात्सर्वप्रयत्नेन योगमेव सदाभ्यसेत् ।

योगाभ्यासो जन्मफलं विफला हि तथा क्रिया ॥१५१॥

tasmātsarvaprayatnena yogameva sadā bhyaset /

yogābhyāso janmaphalaṃ viphalā hi tathā kriyā /151/

Therefore, one should aways make all the efforts to practice yoga. The fruit of one's birth is *yogābhyāsa* (practice of yoga) i.e. we are born here for the practice of yoga. Surely, all life activities become fruitless without yoga practice. -151.

Achieving the Mercy of Mahāmāyā

महामायाप्रसादेन सर्वेषामस्तु तत्सुखम् ।

एतत्सर्वं यथायुक्तं तामेवाराधयेत् ततः ॥१५२॥

mahāmāyāprasādena sarveṣāmastu tatsukham /

etatsarvaṃ yathāyuktaṃ tāmevārādhayet tataḥ /152/

May all gain (the *yogavidyā*) by the mercy of *Mahāmāyā* (the Divine Power). May all be able to achieve the happiness of (*yogavidyā*) in an appropriate way. Therefore, one should properly worship her. -152.

Lord Viṣṇu, The Supreme Jewel of Dedication

यः संस्मृत्या मुनीनामपि दुरितहरो योगसिद्धिप्रदश्च ।

Dattatreya Yogashastra

कारूण्याद्यः प्रवक्ता सुखदुःखसुहृद् योगशास्त्रस्य नाथः ॥१५३॥

तस्याहं भक्तिशुन्योऽप्यखिलजनगुरोः भक्तिचिन्तामणेः हि ।

दत्तात्रेयस्य विष्णोः पदनलिनयुगं नित्यमेव प्रपद्ये ॥१५४॥

yaḥ saṃsmṛtyā munīnāmapi

duritaharo yogasiddhipradaśca /

kārūṇyādyaḥ pravaktā sukhaduḥkha-

suhṛd yogaśāstrasya nāthaḥ /153/

tasyāhaṃ bhaktiśunyo 'pyakhila-

janaguroḥ bhakticintāmaṇeḥ hi /

dattātreyasya viṣṇoḥ padanalina-

yugaṃ nityameva prapadye /154/

I constantly worship the lotus feet of Lord *Viṣṇu* (who incarnated himself) as *Dattātreya*, who destroys all the sins of sages only by recalling him and bestows them all *siddhis* in yoga, who is the primal teacher and lord of *yogaśāstra* and who is compassionate and a friend of all in happiness and suffering. Though I am empty of his devotion, He is the father of all human beings and the supreme jewel of dedication. -153-154.

इति दत्तात्रेय योगशास्त्र ॥

iti dattātreya yogaśāstra //

Thus ends the Dattatreya Yogashastra.

Swami Vishnuswaroop

[62]

Dattatreya Yogashastra

A Key to Transliteration

<u>Vowels</u>

अ आ इ ई उ ऊ ऋ ॠ

a ā i ī u ū ṛ ṝ

लृ ॡ ए ऐ ओ औ अं अः

lṛ lṝ e ai o au aṃ aḥ

<u>Consonants</u>

क ख ग घ ङ - Gutturals:

ka kha ga gha ṅa

च छ ज झ ञ - Palatals:

ca cha ja jha ña

ट ठ ड ढ ण - Cerebrals:

ṭa ṭha ḍa ḍha ṇa

त थ द ध न - Dentals:

ta tha da dha na

प फ ब भ म - Labials:

pa pha ba bha ma

य र ल व - Semivowels:

ya ra la va

श ष स ह - Sibilants:

śa ṣa sa ha

क्ष त्र ज्ञ - Compound Letters:

[63]

[64]

kṣa tra jña

Aspirate: ह - ha, Anusvara: अं - aṃ,

Visharga - aḥ - अः

Unpronounced अ - a - ऽ - ', आ - ā - ऽऽ - ''

Dattatreya Yogashastra

Also by This Author

Yoga Kundalini Upanishad (in English)

Yoga Darshana Upanishad (in English)

Minor Yoga Upanishads (in English)

Hatha Yoga Pradipoka (in English)

Yogatattva Upanishad (in English)

Two Yoga Samhitas (in English)

Triyoga Upanishad (in English)

Gheranda Samhita (in English)

Goraksha Samhita (in English)

Surya Namskara (in Nepali)

Shiva Samhita (in English)

Shiva Samhita (in Nepali)

Durga Strotram (in Nepali)

Vagalamukhi Stotram (in Nepali)

Amogha Shivakavacham (in Nepali)

Copyright© Swami Vishnuswaroop

Swami Vishnuswaroop

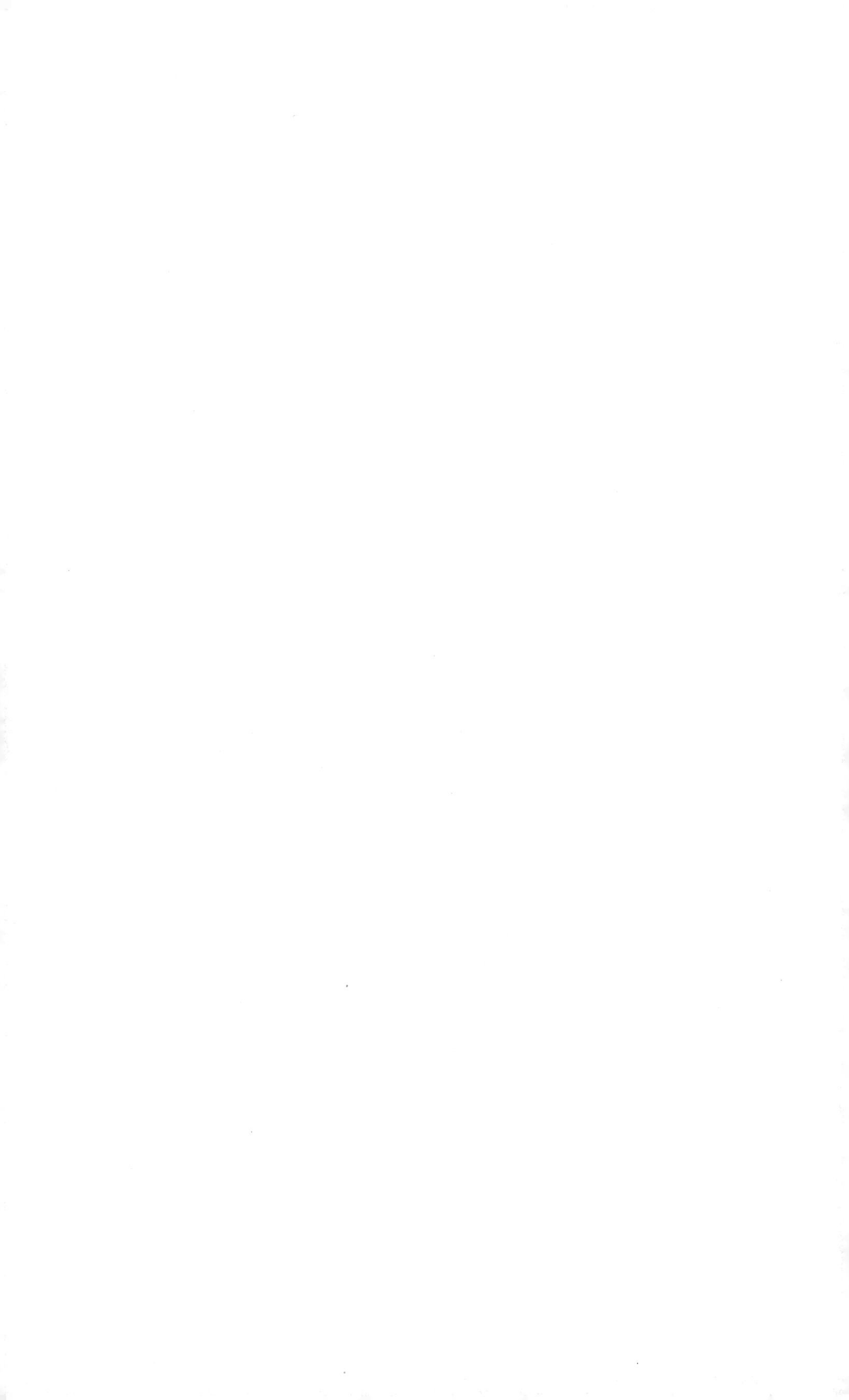